THE DO'S AND DONUTS

Little habits... drastic changes.

With great respect
and looking forward
to cross paths
again. It was a
pleasure to host such
cool person!

TABLE OF CONTENTS

Part I. How to Kick a Deadly Disease Out the Door!

Once upon a time, I was a child eating delicious street junk food after school. I replaced meals with lime sorbet and delicious chips drenched in hot sauce, lime and salt. This went on for who knows how long until one day I became very sick.

My parents took me to the hospital, where I stayed overnight. They said it was typhoid fever and sent me back home. I was fine for a couple of days, but then I was sick again with a high fever that would not go down even after taking several over-the-counter medications. I showered in cold water countless times, but I was still burning in fever. After returning to the hospital for the second time, I was still left without a proper diagnosis.

My parents and I realized it was time to visit the private hospital, however, they too could not find the reason behind my symptoms. Finally, one pediatrician thought I might have lupus and ordered a test in which a large needle was drilled into my sternum to extract a sample of bone marrow. As you can imagine, this was extremely painful. To make matters worse, using anesthesia could compromise my life so they went on without it... it was terrifying. I spent two weeks at the hospital diagnosed with lupus, anemia, kidney infection, and some random amoebas. That junk food must have been delicious!

To put things in perspective, here are some statistics on lupus that you might not know about. The presence of lupus is highest in African people. Only 10% of all lupus patients are men and only 10% of males diagnosed with lupus are children. Hence out of 1.5 million lupus patients in America, only 15 thousand are children[1]. Given the statistics, talk about feeling like Juan in a million! For a while I thought that if I played lottery maybe I could have the same one-in-a-million luck, but I didn't quite make it. What a bummer.

Given the odds of a male child with lupus it is no wonder why doctors could not solve the puzzle. The next step was for my parents to find a doctor who had experience with this disease. Fortunately, we found one relatively close in Monterrey, a city located three hours away from our home.

After the doctor familiarized himself with my case, he prescribed chemotherapy and high doses of prednisone and cortisone plus calcium, multi-vitamin, iron supplements, and for the cherry on top: an Ensure beverage daily. I was a walking cocktail of medications. In addition, my mother made me try every alternative therapy she found including traditional healers, pecan leaf tea, rare teas from South America, chakra healing seminars, meditation, juice therapy, prayer, and the list goes on. It was quite an alternative childhood. My mother would pay me one dollar for every liter of carrot juice I drank, talk about a true health investment!

From my illness, I learned that you can find the positive in any experience. I remember having fun making bets with my father about how many droplets were left in the intravenous chemo solution. I don't know if he let me win on purpose or if he was terrible at guessing, anyhow, I won every time and he would buy me a CD. As strange as it might sound, this made it exciting to get my chemo.

Living through your worst-case scenario also shows you how many people care and support you. Even the owner of the video rental would give my dad free rentals during the time I was in the hospital. People would take me to my favorite restaurants as soon as I was outside of the hospital and able to eat normal food. I felt an incredible amount of love and support from everyone.

When I look back on my memories from this time I cannot remember any pain, as the positive memories are much more vivid. I experienced proof of the human kindness that is hard to notice during everyday life. I remember the positive impact it made to me. To this day, I can attribute this experience as a child as my motivation for giving back to others. Unfortunately, giving so much can be a double-edged sword because some people will take advantage of you. However, I believe that this is their problem and not mine and I continue to open the door for every new friend, and closing a door here and there.

My other key takeaway from this experience is to have faith. Besides all the orthodox treatments I was receiving, I was taken to endless self-healing seminars and workshops. When you are a child it is much easier to believe deeply in something, thus I believed with every cell of my body that I was healing. Interestingly enough, the medical tests started to improve drastically around this time. It surprised both my doctor and the founder of the healing seminars who requested continuous updates on my medical results. I successfully achieved permanent un-medicated remission which is only seen in 7% of all diagnoses lupus cases. What you hold in the core of your beliefs makes a huge difference, **be selective and smart about what you choose to believe.**

Your Attitude Makes a Big Difference

My immune system was attacking my kidneys. As a child, I understood the kidneys worked as filters therefore I decided to rinse my "filters" as much as possible by drinking five liters of water per day. I think the water plus the belief of the water healing me was a powerful duo. Some call it faith, some call it placebo effect, either way it made a crucial difference in my recovery.

Enjoy What You Have

Another challenge was a sodium-free diet. My solution was to put one grain of salt on my tongue, savor as it melted and then take a bite of food. You would be surprised how much flavor you can receive from one grain of salt when you have a heavily restricted diet. Also, breaking up with my love of chips was a challenge. In order to cope with my loss, I would take one of my favorite chips and eat it by the smallest bites in the world, and I really mean the smallest bites in the world. A full bag used to last five minutes in my hands but now one single chip would last ten to fifteen minutes! Although I could only afford to consume one chip, I made sure it was the most delicious-looking chip in the entire bag.

After three years, my health gradually restored. The doctor lowered my medication and suspended chemotherapy. One year later, while I remained on a low dose of medication, my illness stayed in remission. The doctor said it was time to take me off my medication and see if the illness stayed in remission. This was a celebration day; after three years, I finally had freedom from swallowing pills! I must say life felt amazing.

For over fifteen years now, I've been on a permanent un-medicated remission that statistically only about 7% of cases achieve[1]; a rare remission for a rare case of lupus, further continuing my streak of being Juan in a million.

Knowledge is Power

While I was doing my prerequisites for the Physical Therapy degree in college, we had an anatomy and physiology teacher named Ramon de la Torre, who used to rave about teaching us one-third of medical school in two semesters. He was a Patch Adams look-alike and the only gerontologist in the city.

7

Teaching was his passion and he did not care about making a dime from it. Like the all the best teachers do, he shared valuable lessons for life.

Some of these lessons I can immediately recall today, such as:

- "As a health care provider, be humble!"
- "Budget your time!"
- "Vinegar emulsifies fats, use vinegar in your diet."
- "The more you know, the more powerful you are."

I always suggest that my clients empower themselves with knowledge about their health in order to outsmart disease. Recently, I had a client dealing with autoimmune hypothyroidism (Hashimoto). She was taking thyroid hormones T3 and T4 and doing almost everything right except for the fact she was in a "vacation mindset" in Mexico and would drink two margaritas every afternoon. She heard a few times that alcohol would not improve her condition but didn't think it was too important.

I explained that the conversion of T4 into T3 (the bioavailable "usable" form) would take place significantly in the liver and kidneys[2]. If the liver and kidneys had to prioritize detoxifying alcohol, they would likely not process T4 which in effect made taking her medication useless. I was very happy to receive an email from her telling me she had stopped drinking entirely, avoiding situations where a "social" drink might occur. Understanding our biochemistry is the best motivation to adopting a better lifestyle. Your new knowledge unlocks such a positive impact that the previous habits now seem foolish.

Part II. Nature vs. Nurture: Victim or Responsible

We are facing an epidemic of chronic illness. New diseases were bred from our beloved industrial revolution. Mass production of food led the food industry to increase the use of toxic pesticides, antibiotics, and steroids. Also, when we eat animals that are mistreated, we ingest all of their stress hormones. Chefs cook meat under high heat for a "gourmet–seal" unaware of the negative impact this has on health.

We fill our cup of habits by individual drops until eventually we spill over with a chronic disease. Still people believe certain conditions to be "a disease that just happened and nobody knows why." (This was the case with my lupus diagnosis.)

Flavorful Poison

Lovely news! The industry has found a toxic chemical that tastes great and best of all it is cheaper to produce than using real ingredients. It is called monosodium glutamate or MSG.

Meet fibromyalgia, a mysterious disease of the 21st Century. Patients get fatigue and generalized pain in tendons and joints. Doctors press some points in the body, and if they are tender then you get labeled with fibromyalgia! With no explanation of why it happens they label and condemn patients to a chronic degenerative disease, meaning it gets worse with no hope of a cure. There is a case report of four women with fibromyalgia whose symptoms disappeared when they stopped consuming MSG[4].

Go on and savor your MSG with those cramping tendons... lovely! Chinese food? Even better! It is heavily loaded with MSG. People must know the drastic difference these apparently insignificant changes can make. A few days ago, I saw a "gourmet" MSG seasoning at the supermarket. Since when is MSG considered gourmet!?

Where Have All the Nutrients Gone?

In the process of refining wheat the fiber and the minerals necessary for your body to metabolize wheat itself are removed. Also with the removal of fiber, the resulting refined carbohydrates turn into glucose faster, spiking our blood glucose to a dangerous level (untreated high blood sugar can cause blindness) forcing the pancreas to produce insulin immediately to lower it. This glucose ends up being converted into fat for future use... a "future use" that will likely not come. People start becoming 300 pound warehouses of "future use" energy, not to mention *diabetic* due to pancreatic exhaustion. Oh, but it's so darn sweet, isn't it?

Percentage of nutrients lost when wheat flour is refined:

Vitamin	Percentage
Thiamine	77%
Riboflavin	80%
Niacin	81%

Vitamin B6	72%
Pantothenic acid	50%
Folic acid	67%
Vitamin E	86%
Choline	30%

Mineral	Percentage
Magnesium	85%
Potassium	77%
Calcium	60%
Iron	76%
Zinc	78%
Copper	68%
Manganese	86%
Chromium	40%

- Schroeder HA. Losses of vitamins and trace minerals resulting from processing and preservation of foods. American Journal Clinical Nutrition 1971;24:562-573

Now, you may be wondering: why would they commit such a crime removing these nutrients?

First, removing fiber from food makes the food taste sweeter so the sugar crackheads can get their fix. Second, removing the fiber reduces spoilage thereby increasing shelf life. In turn, the food industry kills two birds with one stone, or more like 76,488 birds?

In 2013, 76,488 people died from Diabetes. The war in Iraq killed around 120,000 people in the period from 2003-2013[5]. Diabetes killed in one year, what the war did in 6.3 years! Considering that around 90% of Diabetes cases are Type 2, we can see that Type 2 Diabetes kills more people than war does annually.

COLOR-FULL of $h^t

Another example of a disease brought on by food additives is Carpal Tunnel Syndrome which is caused when nerves of the wrist start pinching leading to numbness and pain from the fingertips all the way to the neck. It is usually triggered by mechanical pressure on the wrist from long hours of computer work and a lack of vitamin B6[6]. Both the food coloring Red 40 and the pesticides used to treat onions greatly impair the body's ability to absorb vitamin B6[7] and resulting in Carpal Tunnel Syndrome.

Other diseases resulting from B6 deficiency include: depression, confusion, anemia and seizures[8-13]. B6 is critical for the synthesis of non-essential amino acids[14]. When referring to amino acids, non-essential means that the body can synthesize them and they are not obligatory in the diet. Ironically, if we can't synthesize them due to lack of B6 they are hence "non-essential," but essential while we're swallowing food coloring and pesticides.

The problem nowadays is that many diets aim for a one-size-fits-all approach. Have you ever tried those one-size-fits-all clothing or accessories? You usually end up with quite loose winter gloves! The same theory exists for dieting. There is no single diet that will work for everybody. Nonetheless, I have not heard one case where Red 40, Yellow 6, or monosodium glutamate has been beneficial to anyone. **Bottom Line:** Food additives enrich the food and pharmaceutical industries pocketbook; unfortunately, your health is not of interest to them.

Simply put, we are victims of habits we willfully choose. You create your own personal heaven or hell based on the food you choose to eat.

Here are some tips that you hear so often that you might be desensitized to them but, nevertheless, these are rules to live by:

1. Eat plenty of green leafy vegetables.

2. Choose fruit for dessert.

3. Do not consume refined-white anything (sugar, rice, bread).

4. Cook food properly, with low heat, and an adequate smoke-point oil. Also use water/humidity such as with a steamer. Adding a tablespoon of water when cooking your food prevents the pan from heating roughly above the water boiling point (100C). Steaming your food will also enhance the food texture, just be aware that it takes a few times to get the right timing so keep an eye on the food.

5. Limit your sodium intake. Beware that processed food is usually loaded with sodium.

6. Only eat one animal protein per meal, do not mix animal proteins. For example, meat and

cheese, eggs and bacon, chicken and bacon, eggs and cheese, etc. It is a load of work for your digestive system. People often load cheese onto their eggs, bacon and sausage; four different animal proteins! Oh, and would you like a glass of chocolate-milk with that? Have fun with your bloating and concert of gas. Your digestive system becomes a disease time-bomb, ticking waiting to explode with either gastritis, Crohn's disease, IBD (Inflammatory Bowel Disease), celiac disease, cancer, leaky gut, and who knows what else!

Part III. Cooking Methods: Grilled Disease

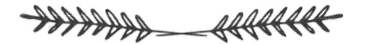

A chronic bad habit is overcooking food as it greatly degrades the longer it is cooked. For example, vitamin C in bell peppers gets spoiled easily. The only exception is tomatoes because although the vitamin C degrades, the lycopene in tomatoes is absorbed much better when cooked[15]. This is due to the fact that trans-lycopene turns into cys-lycopene under heat (the bioavailable form). Tomatoes are one of the few foods containing lycopene, a powerful antioxidant that protects your eyes and prevents certain types of cancer. In this case it is worth sacrificing the vitamin C.

Vegetables high in insoluble fiber can be slightly steamed – such as broccoli, brussel sprouts, and cauliflower – to soften up fiber and ease digestion. Eggplant is also better when cooked fully, as it contains a toxin that is eliminated when cooked. Spinach creates toxins shortly after cooking it[16], so don't leave leftovers. Popeye never left any leftover spinach and neither should you!

The Fountain of Youth! You Can Stop AGEing

Have you ever wondered about the fountain of youth? Why is it that some people age faster than others? One answer is the Advance Glycation End products. They have everything to do with the way we cook food and are the result of proteins and fats bonding with sugars under high heat[17]. AGE is an ironic but perfect acronym because the higher this number, the faster premature aging occurs. High exposure is also linked to some chronic degenerative conditions, such as Type 2 Diabetes, Alzheimer, and osteoarthritis. When you age on the inside, you age on the outside – simple.

Examples of AGE's:

Chicken, 90 g	AGE content (kU)
Oven fried	9,000
Deep fried	6,700

Broiled	5,250
Roasted	4,300
Boiled	1,000
Potatoes, 100 g	**AGE content (kU)**
Boiled 25 minutes	17
Roasted 45 min with 5ml oil	218
French fries, homemade	694
French fries, fast food	1,522
Selected fats, 15 g	**AGE content (kU)**
Butter	3,972
Margarine	2,628
Processed cream cheese	1,632
Breakfast foods	**AGE content (kU)**
Frozen toasted waffle	861
Rice Krispies	600
Frozen toasted pancake	679
Homemade pancake	292
Instant oatmeal	4
Hot dog, 90g	**AGE content (kU)**
Boiled 7 minutes	6,736

Broiled 5 minutes	10,143
Hamburger, 90g	AGE content (kU)
Fried 6 minutes	2,375
McDonalds	4,876
Baby Food, 15 g	AGE content (kU)
Infant formula	487
Breast milk	7

*Goldberg T, Cai W, Peppa M. Advanced glycoxidation end products in commonly consumed foods. J Am Diet Association 2004; 104: 1287-1291.

Every Oil Has Its Personality.

Oils are quite interesting to learn about, they all have different health benefits, but to keep those benefits the oils must be used accordingly to their smoke point. The smoke point is the temperature at which oil starts to burn, losing beneficial properties and producing toxins [18].

Oils with high smoke point are[19]:

Oil	Smoke Point
Avocado	520 F / 271 C

Rice bran	490 F / 254 C
Ghee	485 F / 252 C
Canola (High oleic)	475 F / 246 C
Olive (virgin)	410 F / 210 C
Coconut (unrefined)	350 F / 177 C
Olive (extra virgin)	320 F / 160C

Most vegetables are better steamed than boiled. The water left from steaming/boiling vegetables contains nutrients and you can use it as a base for a salad dressing, risotto, noodles, soup, or stew.

Eggs are better poached, second best option is hard boiled eggs, and the worst choice is to scramble or fry them under high temperature. A healthy scramble option is using chopped tomato and a dash of water on low heat, which will result in eggs that look scrambled, but done with a hint of poaching.

Always cook with a tiny bit of water and low heat. This process takes about the same time when the food is covered and enhances the texture of the food.

For example, placing fish fillets over 1cm slices of tomato, cooking with a teaspoon of apple cider vinegar or water and a tablespoon of oil will leave both tomato and fish melting in your mouth. The best part? You don't even have to flip them, cover them and the vapor gets the job done.

Omegas are the Alphas of Inflammation

Omega-3 is a type of fat (fatty acid) we often associate with fish oil. I find it funny that even the vegan sources such as chia or flaxseed oil taste like fish. I shared a smoothie high in omega-3 with a friend and he told me it reminded him of the cod liver oil that his mother made him drink as a child. So, I guess omega-3 tastes like fish one way or another!

Omega-3 and 6 are the yin and yang of inflammation. Omega-3 fatty acids reduce inflammation while omega-6 fatty acids produce inflammation[20, 21]. While a healthy ratio would be around 8:1, the standard diet has an omega-6 to omega-3 ratio of 16:1[22]. There is nothing radical against omega-6; within balance they maintain metabolism, bone, and reproductive system health. Only when there is excessive amount omega-6 does unhealthy inflammation occur.

Most doctors' visits are inflammation-related. Inflammation must be controlled to prevent health problems including asthma, autoimmune diseases, coronary heart disease, neurodegenerative diseases and many forms of cancer. Additionally, an omega imbalance has been associated with obesity, depression, hyperactivity, irritability, and dyslexia. Next time instead of saying I am sad, angry or anxious, I might say, "I am feeling inflamed!"

The effects of omegas were tested in a prison, and the results linked a high omega-3 diet with a lower incidence of violence[22]. If you are ever arrested, make sure you bring some omega-3 to your cell mate just in case. If the omega-6 to omega-3 ratio is corrected, it is possible to reverse inflammation and its symptoms. A ratio of 2.5:1 reduced cell proliferation in patients with colorectal cancer; a ratio of 3:1 ceased inflammation in patients with rheumatoid arthritis; a ratio of 5:1 was beneficial whereas a 10:1 had negative impact on inflammatory asthma[23]. There are many benefits from fixing an Omega imbalance.

The suffix –*itis* means inflammation... any name rings a bell? A balanced level of Omegas can potentially correct most of the conditions ending in –*itis* such as colitis, arthritis, gastritis, etc.

But that's not all! There are three types of omega-3, and your body cannot just use any, they must be bioavailable.

Omega-3's EPA and DHA, mostly contained in fish, are two forms of omega-3 your body can readily use (they are bioavailable). ALA, the plant-based omega-3, needs to be converted to EPA and DHA[24].

The recommended amount of omega-3 is 300 mg a day[25]. Fish is considered the highest source of omega-3, however, you don't need to eat fish to achieve the recommended value. One portion (15ml) of flaxseed oil gives you at least 200% of the daily recommendation. Some carnivores argue that the omega-3 from vegetable sources don't get the job done as they claim that it is not bioavailable omega-3. Yet, one serving of flaxseed oil contains 7g of omega-3 ALA, from which about 10% (700mg) on average is converted to the bioavailable forms DHA and EPA. So high-five to my vegan friends!

We cannot generalize that all omega-6 fats cause inflammation, there are 11 subtypes of omega-6, and two of them (LA, GLA) have been found to reduce inflammation[26].

Get Your Omegas Balanced Easily:

An easy way to maintain a balanced proportion of omegas is mixing 5 parts olive oil with 1 part of flaxseed oil or chia seed oil. You can add some of your favorite dry herbs or spices and use on salads, soups and dishes. **Do not use this mixture for cooking as it will be sensitive to heat.** Vinegar emulsifies fat, meaning it turns oil into liquid and therefore helps with fat metabolism, absorption and elimination (in theory, due to larger surface area). Adding some organic apple cider vinegar will make a great vinaigrette, plus adding a hint of probiotics.

Not long ago I was teaching a nutritional medicine workshop. While adding apple cider vinegar to guacamole, I mentioned the fact that the benefits are not scientifically proven. Suddenly, one of the students mentioned she met someone who definitely attributed dissolving kidney stones drinking one tablespoon of apple cider vinegar with water every day. Right then and there I said: "Okay, now that we have proof, let's add some extra!" splashing a few extra squirts from the bottle, friendly laughter followed.

Part IV. Tired of Being Tired... of Being Tired

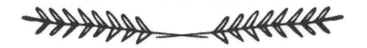

What makes us chronically tired? It would be great to have one single answer, however, tiredness is caused by many factors – lack of stress hormones, low blood sugar or insulin, improper sleep hygiene, or reactive hypoglycemia – luckily, all of these can be corrected with proper lifestyle changes.

Meet Hypoglycemia

The word hypoglycemia is derived from three parts. From *hypo* meaning below, *glykys* meaning sweet, and *haima* for blood; hence quite literally translates to low blood sugar. Besides people on a strict ketogenic diet, Glucose is what most people use to produce energy. Sugar is transformed to adenosine triphosphate (ATP), the form of energy your cells use.

For those diagnosed with Type 2 Diabetes, some might have enough blood sugar but not enough insulin to metabolize it, while others might have developed a resistance to insulin. In both cases, patients often lack energy due to low blood sugar, high in the blood but low inside the cells.

If there is insulin resistance in the brain there may be risk for Alzheimer's, it is even referred to as Type 3 diabetes [27]. People with Type 2 diabetes are said to have a 50% to 65% greater chance of developing Alzheimer's. This is evidenced by research that shows deposits of a protein (amyloid beta) in the pancreas, the same protein deposits found in the brain of Alzheimer patients[28].

Diabetes Cured?

My mother and her husband came to visit after they had been told by two doctors that his pancreas was no longer working. The doctors said, "Just take the little pill and do not worry about your diet." I informed him about the effects of refined carbs on his pancreas, blood glucose and insulin levels. I also told him about the minerals needed to metabolize sugar such as magnesium, chromium, and copper. During their ten day stay, I created a nutritional meal plan that consisted of probiotic food such as sauerkraut, zucchini relish, kombucha, water kefir, and even some shrimp cocktail using probiotic ketchup.

I told him, if a car was running on the first and second gear several months, the transmission will eventually break down from such forced use. The same thing happens when you force the pancreas to produce high amounts of insulin all the time to regulate your sugar-crackhead indulgence. The point when your pancreas "machine" no longer produces enough insulin to lower sugar, or you overuse insulin cell receptors, you may be forced to pick up some unfriendly hitchhikers like Diabetes and Alzheimer.

I suggested 40mg magnesium orotate in the morning; 100mcg GTF (glucose tolerance factor) chromium after breakfast, 500mg acerola berry powder twice a day for natural vitamin C, and 9.5 mg of Zinc orotate after lunch (zinc and magnesium separately). His blood sugar has been stable for over year.

He is a smart guy with good reasoning. I told him: "You can live the next five years indulging in harmful foods you love, and the next five suffering or the next ten years enjoying life but with some dietary restrictions. It is your call, but you cannot say nobody warned you about consequences...." By the way, I clarified that saying he was living only ten more years was just a practical metaphor! There was a funny moment during a meal when my mother offered him a piece of white bread or a sip of soda and he refused radically. To ease the awkward silence, I jokingly suggested that my mother must have bought him life insurance that she was eager to collect on.

Meet Hypoadrenalism: I Want My Stress Back

Hypoadrenalism is the inability to produce cortisol (the stress hormone) possibly due to an overused adrenal gland. Tame your stress now because you might need it in the future to maintain a healthy energy level. In order to produce cortisol, the pituitary gland first needs to release adrenocorticotropic hormones (ACTH). Since adrenal function is rooted in the pituitary gland, **a good practice is to use fluoride-free toothpaste, as fluoride is believed to "calcify" the pituitary**. Although cholesterol has been tagged as our enemy, it is essential to produce stress hormones (cortisol, epinephrine, norepinephrine, and adrenaline). Keep a balance.

Hypoadrenalism may be autoimmune, meaning the immune system attacks the adrenal glands to the point where they no longer work properly. Unfortunately, usually when it shows clinical signs the glands are already 80% damaged[29].

The body is always trying to maintain balance (homeostasis). When blood sugar levels fall, the adrenal glands release adrenaline to compensate for energy, resulting in anxiety, panic, palpitations, sweating, tremors and abdominal pain.

If you don´t have this discharge of adrenaline, you may suffer from neuroglycopenia (shortage of glucose in the brain), which produces confusion, headache, fatigue, blurred vision, impaired memory, seizures, unconsciousness, personality changes, irritability... and the list goes on. Unfortunately, some people get the two-for-one deal and experience symptoms both of adrenaline response and neuroglycopenia; sounds like being in a horror movie with a hangover.

Live in the Moment

This common philosophy does not apply here! Some people have sugar and refined carb cravings and eating them provides temporary relief, but it is followed by a rebound craving that leads to overeating and obesity. When this happens refined carbs and sugar turn into glucose rapidly. Since the body does not need such high glucose for ATP/energy, the excess is transformed into fat for energy storage by an enzyme stimulated by insulin. My anatomy teacher explained the breakdown of complex carbs by the amylase in your saliva saying, "I have an experiment for you: try chewing cooked potato without butter or anything, it will taste horrible, like it is not meant to be eaten like that, but keep chewing and it will taste sweet as complex carbs brake down into simple sugars." I get nostalgia over those school days.

Fatigued for TOO Long

Your fatigue is considered "chronic" if it lasts longer than six months without a reason and it is accompanied by four or more of the following symptoms:

- Sore throat
- Impaired short-term memory
- Tender lymph nodes
- Muscle pain
- Joint pain without swelling or redness
- Un-refreshing sleep
- Headaches of a new kind
- Post-exercise malaise longer than 24 hours
- Epstein-Barr, also known as mononucleosis or "kiss disease" can create chronic fatigue.

* Gaby AR. Nutritional Medicine 2011. Chronic Fatigue Syndrome; 326:1233.

*Note that for hypoglycemia, hypoadrenalism, diabetes, insulin resistance, there is a test you need to take. Consult your doctor.

Suggestions for an Uplifted Energy:

Sweet ain't really sweet! The utmost important thing for chronic fatigue is to stop overeating sugar. Beware that even if you don't directly add sugar to your food, high amounts are added to many commercial products (ketchup, cereals, soft drinks, etc.) with nicknames to deceive you (dextrose, sucrose, fructose, maltodextrin, corn syrup, cane juice, barley malt, etc.). Also, eating refined carbs such as white bread is a triple threat for you. Glucose crackheads be all like: "Triple treat yay! A sweet, chewy, dopamine dose!"

Indeed a triple threat:

- It converts rapidly into glucose and subsequently into fat storage.
- Lack of fiber speeds up the glucose spike.
- Last but not least, flour refining removes approximately 70% of vitamins and

minerals, including magnesium and chromium[30] which are essential for glucose metabolism:

No refined carbs. If you do consume refined carbs combine them with some almonds or anything rich in fiber to buffer the glucose spike.

Eat small meals with enough protein. This is especially important for vegetarians and vegans. Combine foods that complete the nine essential amino acids, not particularly in the same meal, but on a daily basis. An example of a complete protein combo would be rice and beans.

Eat smart snacks like dried fruit and nuts. When your glucose crackhead cells are craving sugar and fat, your mind translates that into candy and pizza. (Hopefully not candied pizza! A.K.A. donuts, my biggest Donut for you!) If you feed your stomach sugar from dried fruits and healthy fats from nuts, your body gets a dose of fat and sugar and you stop craving the unhealthy options. A good option is Brazil nuts, which contain magnesium and high amounts of selenium, both good for regulating sugar. But beware that only 6 Brazil nuts contain about 700% of selenium.

Include them in a nut mix to avoid overeating. Cashews are also a good option; they contain the nine essential amino acids.

High protein and complex carbohydrates. They can treat low blood sugar as complex carbs are absorbed slowly and can maintain your glucose level (aim for a low glycemic index). Protein helps regulate blood sugar as amino acids serve as raw material to create new glucose (gluconeogenesis). It also helps to consume six small meals per day or have some smart snacks between meals.

Avoid coffee, alcohol and sugar. If you cannot avoid coffee, replace it with a lighter stimulant such as green tea. Alcohol inhibits energy production (gluconeogenesis), limit your alcohol intake or better yet, avoid it altogether. Intrinsic sugars, such as those contained in fruit are fine in moderation but stay away from artificial fructose.

Opioid peptides. They are short-chain amino acid molecules, which have an opium-like effect. The body produces opioid peptides called endorphins, often called "the happiness hormone." Opioid peptides can improve plasma insulin, nonetheless, most of these peptides are found in allergenic foods such as soy, milk, rye, barley, and gluten. Luckily, they are found in spinach as well, which is a great nutrient-dense food. These peptides and not tryptophan* might be the reason why a glass of milk might help induce sleep. Opioid peptides also regulate food intake, emotional balance and motivation.

*Tryptophan competes with a handful of other amino acids to cross the blood brain barrier, and it loses efficacy when taken with protein. If you supplement tryptophan you should take it after eating some cereal such as oatmeal.

Identify possible reactive hypoglycemia or food allergy. Both can cause fatigue, and you can identify them as follow:

<u>Flu-like symptoms</u>: caused by wheat, milk, beef, tomato, pineapple, pumpkin.

<u>Fatigue symptoms</u>: caused by sugar, refined grains, wheat, corn, rice.

Supplements to consider for fatigue:

1. Chromium: 200mcg/day of chromium (polynicotinate) was found helpful for chronic fatigue. A study that used 500-1000mg of

chromium per day for 12 weeks resulted in improvements for low blood sugar [31]. However, chromium must be avoided or carefully administered by your physician, especially if you have a history of diabetes, kidney disease, liver disease, clinical depression, anxiety, or schizophrenia.

2. Magnesium: 340mg/day of magnesium ingestion improved low blood sugar in a double-blind study (57% vs. 25% placebo)[32]. In another study, 80% of patients receiving magnesium reported having more energy, a better emotional state, and less pain [33]. Recently the German doctor Hans Nieper discovered that orotic acid increased bioavailability of some minerals. This finding showed that magnesium orotate it is one of the best options to treat fatigue. Mg Citrate is the least bioavailable and almost useless. Magnesium is needed for ATP synthesis, the form of energy in the body. It is okay to take magnesium on an empty stomach, but if stomach uneasiness occurs, take it with food. Magnesium must be used with caution if you have a history of kidney disease.

Note on blood testing: Mg might appear normal in blood, but there might be an inability to transport Mg from serum into cells. This was noted by doing a large blood infusion of Magnesium and noticing the percentage retained and eliminated then by estimating the deficiency accordingly[34]. Something similar happens with B12; it was found in the low/normal range in blood but nonetheless it was undetectable in the cerebrospinal fluid. This indicates either an impaired ability to transport B12 through the blood brain barrier or that the B12 was breaking down before reaching the nervous system[35]. Blood testing is not always the answer.

Conclusion

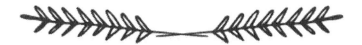

Writing a book is a lot more work than I imagined, I estimated 3 weeks for this little guide and it has been 18 months in the making. Also making nutritional medicine entertaining is quite a challenge; hence I had to break this book down in two parts before my own life broke in ten.

Healing yourself is a lifetime journey. There are many people and philosophies that may help you. Please visit my website www.lifesynergyretreat.com and my blogs civilianpsychology.com and healingbolus.com if you would like help in determining your next step or need a resource of hope. After more than fifteen years of living with lupus, I remain happy and grateful to say that I maintain my health completely through food, knowledge and personal awareness.

What I ask, is for you to be aware of your choices; to stop being a puppet of mass media, to read your food labels, and to be informed. Ignorance is not bliss when it comes to losing your health. Health is the one most precious thing in life, without it even if you have a great career, money, the love of your life, and a great family, you will likely not be able to fully enjoy. Make your health your first priority and live accordingly. Mental health is just as important, treat your mind like you treat your body and take care of both. If you are feeling tortured while resisting a scoop of ice-cream, give it to yourself as a treat; it is the daily bad habits that harm you the most, not a random treat. I hope from the bottom of my heart this improves your lifestyle and helps you avoid going through the pain of a chronic or auto-immune disorder.

I would love to hear from you:
contact@lifesynergyretreat.com

For information on holistic retreats please visit:
www.lifesynergyretreat.com

You are welcome to visit our blogs:
www.healingbolus.com
www.civilianpsychology.com

Bibliography

Alexander JC. Chemical and Biological properties related to toxicity of heated fats. J Toxicol Environ Health 1981; 7: 125- 138.

Anderson RA, Polansky MM, Bryden NA, et al. Effects of supplemental chromium on patients with symptoms of reactive hypoglycemia. Metabolism 1987; 36:351-355.

Anonymous. Cerebral spinal fluid vitamin B12 deficiency in CFS. CFIDS chronicle 1997 (Winter):57.

Bapurao S, Raman L, Tulpule PG. Biochemical assessment of vitamin B6 nutritional status on pregnant women with orolingual manifestations. Am J Clin Nutr 1982; 36: 581- 586.

Boileau, AC, et al. "Cis-Lycopene Is More Bioavailable than Trans-Lycopene in Vitro and in Vivo in Lymph-Cannulated Ferrets." *National Center for Biotechnology Information*, U.S. National Library of Medicine, June 1999.

Chhabra, Namrata. "Role of B6 Phosphate in Amino Acid Metabolism." *LinkedIn SlideShare*, LinkedIn Corporation, 12 July 2012.

Childers NF, Russo GM. The Nightshades and Health. Somerville, NJ, Horticultural Publications, Somerset Press, Inc.,1977.

Cox IM, Campbell MJ, Dowson D. red blood cell magnesium and chronic fatigue syndrome. Lancet 1991; 337:757-760.

de la Monte, Suzanne M., and Jack R. Wands. "Alzheimer's Disease Is Type 3 Diabetes–Evidence Reviewed." *National Center for Biotechnology Information*, U.S. National Library of Medicine, Nov. 2008.

de Lorgeril M, Salen P. New insights into the health effects of dietary saturated and omega-6 and omega-3 polyunsaturated fatty acids. BMC Med. 2012; 10:50.

"Diabetes." *Centers for Disease Control and Prevention*, U.S. Department of Health & Human Services, 3 May 2017.

"Do You Have a T4 to T3 Conversion Problem?" *Natural Endocrine Solutions*, Natural Endocrine Solutions.

E.J. Phillips. J. Agric. Food Chem., 1968, 16 (1), pp 88–91.

Folkers K, Wolaniuk A, Vadhanavikit S. Enzymology of the response of the carpal tunnel syndrome and need for determination of the RDAs for vitamins B6 and B2 for disease states. Ann N Y Acad Sci 1990; 585:295-301.

Gaby AR. Nutritional Medicine 2011. Cooking and Storage of Foods; 5:15.

Gaby AR. Nutritional Medicine 2011. Omega – 3 Fatty Acids; 66:227.

Gaby AR. The Doctor's guide to vitamin B6. Emmaus, PA, Rodale Press, 1984.

Harvard Health Publishing. "Why Not Flaxseed Oil?" *Harvard Health Publishing*, Harvard University, Oct. 2006.

Hawkins WW, Barsky J. An experiment on human vitamin B6 deprivation. Science 1948; 208: 284-286.

Holland-Frei. Cancer Medicine (2010). Complications of Cancer and Their Treatment, Adrenal Insufficiency. 37; 1906.

Kapoor, R, and YS Huang. "Gamma Linolenic Acid: an Antiinflammatory Omega-6 Fatty Acid." National Center for Biotechnology Information, U.S. National Library of Medicine, Dec. 2006.

Liu, Chia-Chen, et al. "Apolipoprotein E and Alzheimer Disease: Risk, Mechanisms, and Therapy." *National Center for Biotechnology Information*, U.S. National Library of Medicine, 8 Jan. 2013.

"Lupus Facts and Statistics." *The National Resource Center on Lupus*, Lupus Foundation of America, 30 Oct. 2017.

Manuel y Keenoy B, Moorkens G, Vertommen J, et al. Magnesium status and parameters of the oxidant-antioxidant balance in patients with chronic fatigue: effects of supplementation with magnesium. J Am Coll Nutr 2000;19: 374-382.

Meydani SN, Ribaya – Mercado JD, Russell RM, et al. Vitamin B6 deficiency impairs interleukin 2 production and lymphocyte proliferation in elderly adults. Am J Clin Nutr 1991;53: 1275-1280.

Meyer, Barbara J., et al. "Baseline Omega-3 Index Correlates with Aggressive and Attention Deficit Disorder Behaviours in Adult Prisoners." *National Center for Biotechnology Information*, U.S. National Library of Medicine, 20 Mar. 2015.

Mueller JF, Vilter RW. Pyridoxine deficiency in human beings induced with deoxypyridoxine. J Clin Invest 1950; 29: 193-201.

Schroeder HA. Losses of vitamins and trace minerals resulting from processing and preservation of foods. American Journal Clinical Nutrition 1971; 24:562-573.

Simopoulos, AP. "The Importance of the Ratio of Omega-6/Omega-3 Essential Fatty Acids." *National Center for Biotechnology Information*, U.S. National Library of Medicine, Oct. 2002.

Smith JD, Terpening CM, Schmidt SOF, Gums JG. Relief of fibromyalgia symptoms following discontinuation of dietary excitotoxins. Ann Pharmacother 2001; 35:702-706.

Spies TD, Bean WB, Ashe WF. A note on the use of vitamin B6 in human nutrition. JAMA 1939; 112: 2414-2415.

Stebbing JB, Turner MO, Franz KB. Reactive hypoglycemia and magnesium. Magnesium Bull 1982; 2:131-134.

The Culinary Institute of America (1996). The New Professional Chef (6th edition ed.). John Wiley & Sons.

Walsh, Nancy. "Prolonged Remission Now Possible in Lupus." *MedPage Today*, MedPage Today, LLC, 2 Aug. 2015.

Made in the USA
Columbia, SC
24 October 2020

23352532R00036